THE KIDNEY-BOOSTING DIET

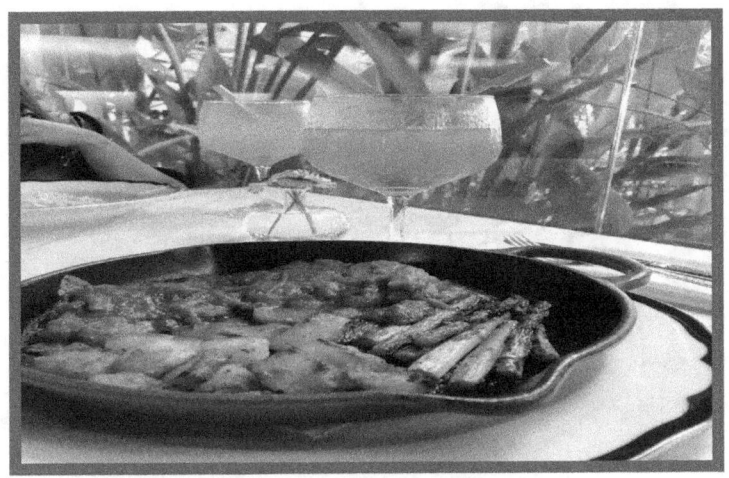

FOODS TO SUPPORT YOUR RENAL FUNCTION

BY

JOYFUL BOFEST

COPYRIGHT

TABLE OF CONTENTS

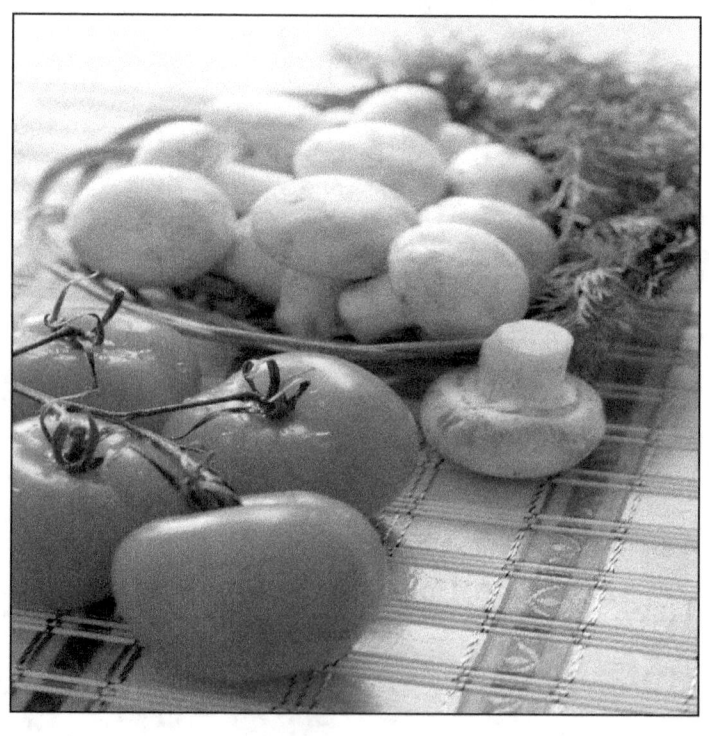

INTRODUCTION:

In the complex orchestra of bodily functions, our kidneys play a vital symphony. These two bean-shaped organs, located in our lower back, are unsung heroes, tirelessly filtering waste and toxins from our blood. However, in the hustle and bustle of modern life, we often neglect their health. A kidney-stimulating diet appears to be the guiding light for optimal kidney health. This comprehensive guide aims to provide you with the knowledge and options to support your kidney function naturally. It introduces a balanced approach to nutrition, emphasizing foods that nourish and restore these remarkable organs. From nutrient-dense vegetables to hydration strategies, each chapter is designed to give you practical, actionable steps.

Join us on this journey to discover a balanced diet that not only protects your kidneys but also enhances your overall health. Together, let's build a resilient foundation for vibrant, healthy lives.

Chapter 1:Important role of kidneys. Before going into details about a kidney-boosting diet, it is important to understand the essential role these organs play in maintaining our health. In addition to filtering, the kidneys also regulate blood pressure, balance electrolytes, and produce essential hormones. This chapter provides a clear and accessible overview, laying the foundation for your journey toward better kidney health.

Chapter 2: Nourish nephrons. In this section, we explore the many nutrient-rich foods that form the foundation of our approach to enhancing kidney function. From brightly colored fruits to lean proteins, we highlight the key players in supporting and restoring kidney function. Discover how simple changes to your diet can have a profound impact on kidney health and vitality.

Chapter 3: Hydration and kidney health. Hydration is often underestimated but is of great importance for kidney function. Adequate fluid intake ensures the kidneys can effectively filter waste and maintain electrolyte balance. This chapter provides practical strategies for staying well hydrated, guiding you through a balanced approach to optimizing your kidney health.

Chapter 4:Stay away from harmful culprits. Incorporating beneficial foods is just as important as recognizing and avoiding foods that can strain our kidneys. This section highlights common nutritional factors that can affect optimal kidney function. By understanding these potential pitfalls, you will be better equipped to make informed choices for your kidney health.

Chapter 5:Tips for kidney health care.

Putting theory into practice, this chapter offers a selection of delicious recipes that stimulate the kidneys. From satisfying main courses to refreshing drinks, each recipe is carefully crafted to maximize nutritional benefits while stimulating your taste buds. These culinary creations make a kidney-boosting diet a delicious and enjoyable experience.

Conclusion: Journey to vibrant kidney health. At the end of this guide, you're armed with a wealth of knowledge and practical steps to begin your journey of change to healthy kidney health. The kidney-boosting diet is more than just a dietary approach; It's a commitment to nurturing and honoring the important role your kidneys play in your overall health.

Follow this path with confidence, knowing that you hold the power to improve and save your kidney function. With dedication and thoughtful choices, you pave the way to a future filled with vitality and resilience.

I hope you find this next section helpful! Let me know if there's anything else you'd like to add or change.

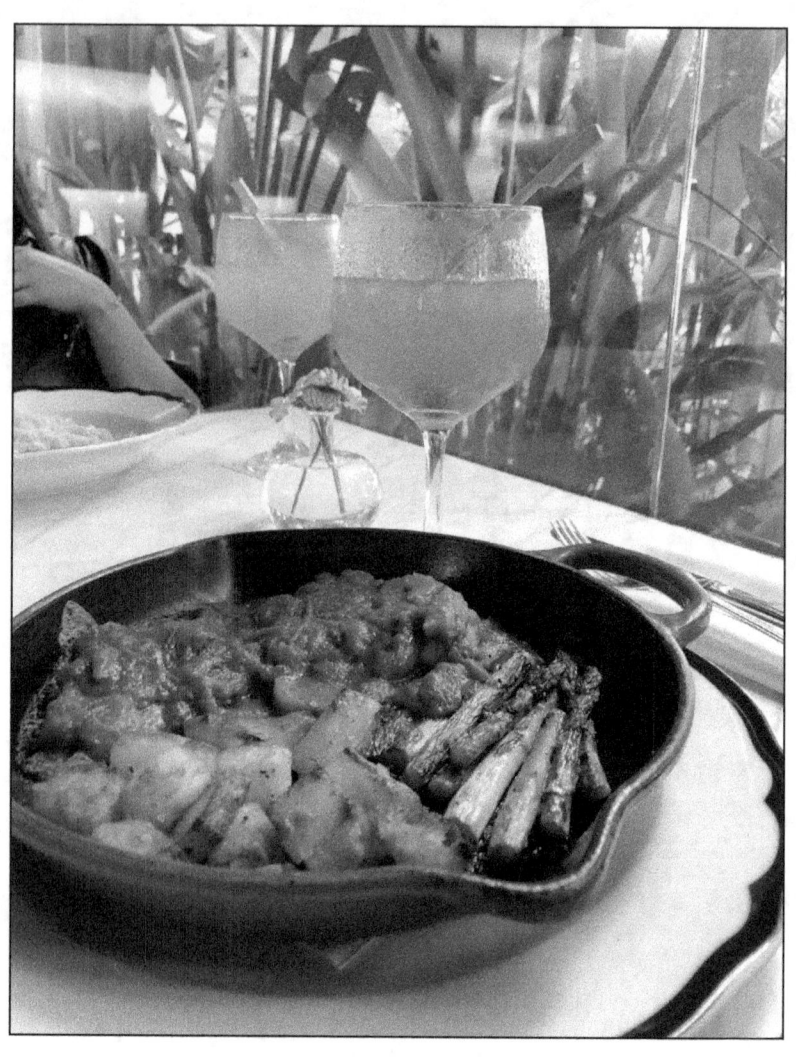

CHAPTER ONE:
THE KIDNEY'S CRUCIAL ROLE

The kidneys play a vital role in the body by filtering waste, regulating various physiological parameters, maintaining electrolyte and acid-base balance, controlling blood pressure, producing red blood cells, activating vitamin D, and aiding in detoxification processes. These functions are crucial for overall health and bodily homeostasis

The kidneys are essential organs responsible for filtering waste products from the blood and excreting them as urine. They also help regulate blood pressure, electrolyte levels, and pH balance. Additionally, the kidneys play a role in producing red blood cells, activating vitamin D, and aiding in the detoxification of harmful substances. These functions collectively contribute to the body's overall well-being and proper functioning.

ROLES OF KIDNEY IN THE BODY

1. **Filtration:** The kidneys filter blood to remove waste products, excess substances (like salts and water), and toxins. This process occurs in tiny units called nephrons.

2. **Excretion:** After filtration, the kidneys excrete the filtered waste products as urine. Urine contains water, salts, and other waste materials that the body needs to eliminate.

3. **Regulation:** The kidneys help regulate various physiological parameters such as blood pressure, electrolyte levels, and pH (acidity or alkalinity) in the body.

4. **Blood pressure:** The kidneys help control blood pressure by adjusting the volume of blood and the concentration of certain electrolytes in the bloodstream. They do this through a combination of hormonal signals and filtration processes.

5. **Electrolyte balance:** Electrolytes are minerals that carry an electric charge. The kidneys maintain the balance of electrolytes like sodium, potassium, calcium, and phosphate in the body, which is crucial for proper cellular function.

6. **Acid-base balance:** The kidneys help regulate the body's pH level, ensuring it remains within a narrow range for optimal cellular function. They

do this by excreting hydrogen ions and reabsorbing bicarbonate ions.

7. **Erythropoiesis:** The kidneys produce and release a hormone called erythropoietin in response to low oxygen levels. This hormone stimulates the production of red blood cells in the bone marrow.

8. **Renin-angiotensin system:** The kidneys release the enzyme renin, which is part of a complex system that helps regulate blood pressure and fluid balance in the body.

9. **Metabolism of vitamin D:** The kidneys convert inactive vitamin D into its active form, which is necessary for the absorption of calcium and

phosphate in the intestines. This is crucial for maintaining strong bones.

10. **Detoxification:** The kidneys play a crucial role in detoxifying the body by filtering out harmful substances like drugs, chemicals, and metabolic waste products.

11. Reabsorption: After filtration, the nephron reabsorbs essential substances like glucose, amino acids, and certain ions back into the bloodstream. This ensures that valuable nutrients are not lost in the urine.

12. **Secretion:** The nephron also secretes additional waste products and ions into the urine, further fine-tuning the

These functions collectively ensure that the body maintains a stable internal environment, allowing cells to function optimally. The kidneys are indispensable for overall health and well-being.

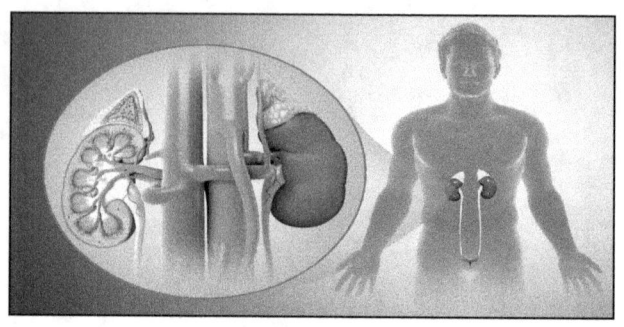

THE NEPHRON CARRIES OUT SEVERAL VITAL FUNCTIONS:

Nephrons are the functional units of the kidneys, responsible for the filtration of blood and the formation of urine. They are tiny, complex structures located within the kidneys. Each kidney contains thousands of nephrons, making them the essential components of the kidney's filtration system.

Nourishing the nephrons is a crucial aspect of maintaining optimal kidney health. The nephrons are the microscopic filtering units within the kidneys responsible for regulating the composition of the blood and eliminating waste products. To ensure their proper function, it's essential to adopt a balanced and kidney-friendly diet.

One of the key elements in nourishing the nephrons is controlling sodium intake. Excessive sodium can lead to high blood pressure, which can strain the delicate filtration process in the nephrons. Therefore, it's advisable to limit the consumption of high-sodium foods like processed snacks, canned goods, and certain condiments.

Additionally, incorporating foods rich in antioxidants can be beneficial. Antioxidants help protect the nephrons from oxidative stress, which can damage their delicate structures. Fruits and vegetables, particularly those vibrant in color like berries, spinach, and carrots, are excellent sources of antioxidants.

Maintaining proper hydration is another vital aspect. Ample water intake ensures that the nephrons have enough fluid to facilitate the filtration process effectively. It helps in flushing out waste products and toxins from the body. However, it's important to strike a balance, as excessive fluid intake can strain the kidneys.

Balanced protein consumption is also crucial for nephron health. While protein is essential for bodily functions, excessive intake can put strain on the kidneys. Opting for lean protein sources like poultry, fish, and plant-based alternatives can help maintain a healthy balance.

Moreover, keeping an eye on potassium levels is important. The kidneys play a significant role in regulating potassium levels in the body. Foods rich in potassium, such as bananas, oranges, and potatoes, should be consumed in moderation, especially for individuals with kidney conditions.

Lastly, it's imperative to limit the intake of phosphorus-rich foods. Elevated phosphorus levels can disrupt the mineral balance in the body, leading to complications for the nephrons. Foods like dairy products, nuts, and certain processed foods are high in phosphorus and should be consumed judiciously.

In conclusion, nourishing the nephrons involves adopting a well-rounded and kidney-friendly diet. This includes controlling sodium intake, incorporating antioxidant-rich foods, maintaining proper hydration, balancing protein consumption, monitoring potassium levels, and limiting phosphorus-rich foods. By paying attention to these dietary considerations, one can support optimal kidney health and ensure the nephrons function effectively in filtering waste and maintaining bodily homeostasis.

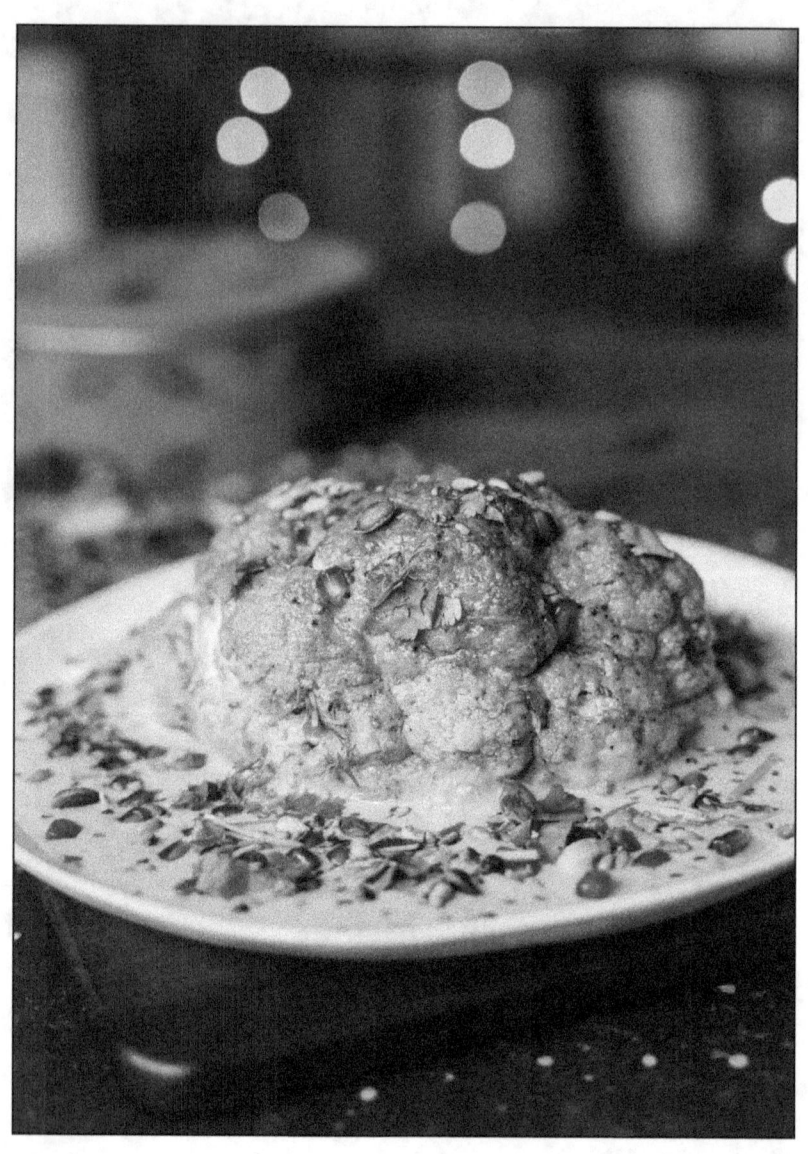

CHAPTER 3:

HYDRATION AND KIDNEY HEALTH

HYDRATION:

1. Water Intake:

The primary component of hydration is water. It is essential for various bodily functions, including digestion, temperature regulation, and waste removal.

2. Electrolytes:

Electrolytes like sodium, potassium, calcium, and magnesium help maintain the balance of fluids in and around your cells. They play a crucial role in muscle function, nerve signaling, and maintaining proper hydration levels.

3. Fluid-Rich Foods:

Fruits and vegetables with high water content, like cucumbers, watermelon, and lettuce, can contribute to overall hydration.

4. Avoiding Dehydrating Beverages:

Beverages like alcohol and caffeinated drinks can lead to increased fluid loss, so moderation is key.

5. Monitoring Urine Color:

It's a simple way to gauge your hydration status. Light-colored urine generally indicates good hydration, while dark-colored urine may suggest dehydration.

KIDNEY HEALTH:

1. **Proper Fluid Balance:** Maintaining the right amount of fluids in the body is crucial for kidney health. Too much or too little can put stress on the kidneys.

2. **Balanced Diet:** A diet rich in fruits, vegetables, whole grains, and lean proteins provides essential nutrients while minimizing the risk of kidney stones and other issues.

3. **Limiting Sodium Intake:** Excessive sodium can lead to high blood pressure and kidney damage. It's recommended to keep sodium intake within a healthy range.

4. **Regular Physical Activity:** Exercise promotes overall health, including cardiovascular health, which indirectly supports kidney function.

5. **Blood Pressure Management:** High blood pressure is a leading cause of kidney problems. Monitoring blood pressure and taking steps to keep it within a healthy range is vital.

6. **Avoiding Smoking and Excessive Alcohol Consumption:** Smoking and heavy alcohol use can contribute to kidney damage and should be avoided.

7. **Regular Health Check-ups:** Routine check-ups with a healthcare provider can help identify any early signs of kidney problems.

8. **Avoiding Overuse of Pain Medications:** Some over-the-counter pain medications, when used excessively, can lead to kidney damage. It's important to follow recommended dosages.

9. **Individual Needs:** The amount of water needed can vary depending on factors like age, activity level, climate, and overall health. Tailor your hydration habits to meet your specific requirements.

10. **Hydration Timing:** Sipping water consistently throughout the day is often more effective than trying to compensate for dehydration all at once.

11. **Hydration During Exercise:** During physical activity, it's crucial to replenish lost fluids. Sports

drinks containing electrolytes can be beneficial for more prolonged and intense workouts.

12. **Monitoring Thirst -** Thirst is a natural signal from your body indicating a need for fluids. Pay attention to it and respond promptly.

13. **Adequate Rest and Stress Management:** Getting enough rest and managing stress levels are essential for overall health, including kidney function. Chronic stress can impact blood pressure and indirectly affect the kidneys.

14. **Diabetes Management:-** If you have diabetes, controlling blood sugar levels is crucial in preventing kidney damage. Regular monitoring and following your healthcare provider's advice is vital.

15. **Regular Blood Sugar and Kidney Function Tests:**- For individuals with diabetes or a family history of kidney disease, routine tests to monitor blood sugar levels and kidney function are crucial for early detection and management.

16. **Avoiding Excessive Protein Intake:** While protein is an essential nutrient, excessive consumption can strain the kidneys, especially for individuals with pre-existing kidney conditions.

17. **Managing Chronic Conditions:** Conditions like high blood pressure and cardiovascular disease can contribute to kidney issues. Managing these conditions with the help of healthcare professionals is crucial.

18. **Avoiding Excessive Use of NSAIDs:** Non-steroidal anti-inflammatory drugs (NSAIDs) like ibuprofen can put extra strain on the kidneys if used excessively. Consult a healthcare provider for suitable alternatives if you need pain relief.

19. **Prompt Medical Attention for Kidney Infections or Stones:** Kidney infections and stones can lead to serious complications if not promptly addressed. Seek medical attention if you experience symptoms like severe pain, fever, or blood in the urine.

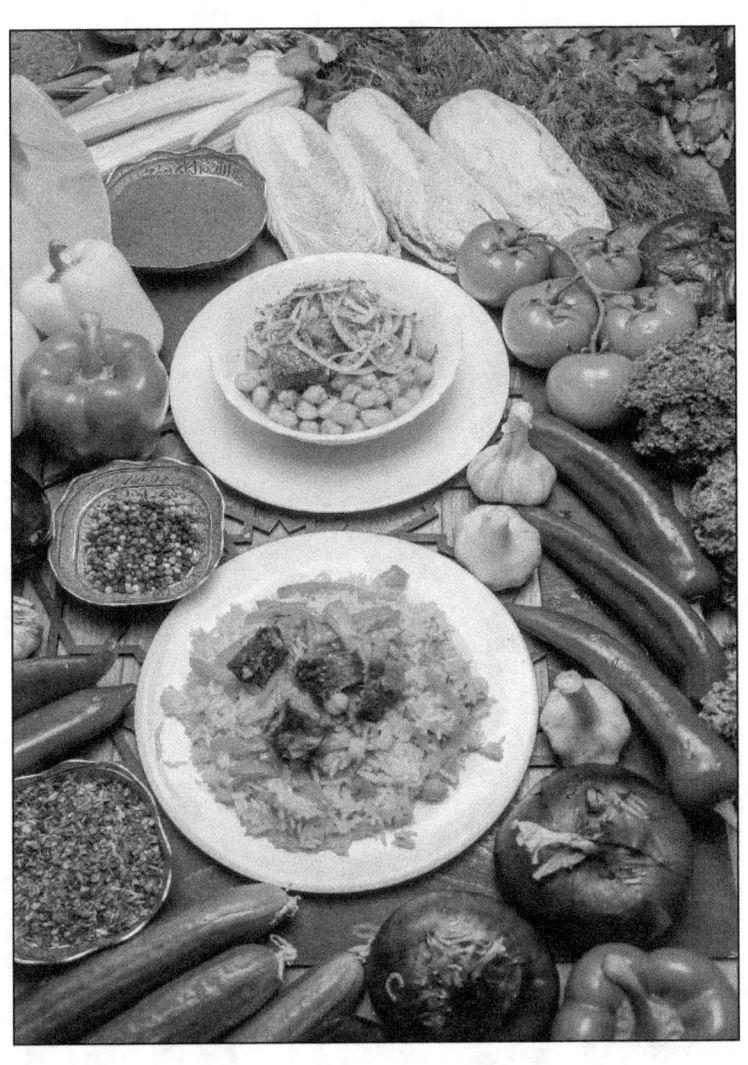

CHAPTER 4:

AVOIDING HARMFUL CULPRITS

1. **Trans Fats:** Risk of heart disease, high cholesterol levels.

2. **Processed Foods** (high in refined sugars, preservatives, and artificial additives): Obesity, diabetes, digestive issues, nutrient deficiencies.

3. **High-Sugar Foods and Beverages:** Obesity, diabetes, tooth decay, inflammation, increased risk of heart disease.

4. **Sugary Drinks** (sodas, energy drinks, fruit juices with added sugars): Weight gain, type 2 diabetes, dental problems, increased risk of chronic diseases.

5. **Artificial Sweeteners** (aspartame, saccharin, sucralose): Potential negative effects on gut health, may disrupt metabolic processes.

6. **Processed Meats** (hot dogs, sausages, deli meats): Increased risk of heart disease, cancer (especially colorectal cancer).

7. **Excessive Salt/Sodium:** High blood pressure, kidney problems, increased risk of stroke.

8. **Highly Processed Grains** (white bread, white rice, sugary cereals): Rapid blood sugar spikes, weight gain, nutrient deficiencies.

9. **Artificial Trans Fats** (partially hydrogenated oils): Increases bad cholesterol levels, risk of heart disease.

10. **Highly Caffeinated Drinks** (energy drinks, excessive coffee): Sleep disturbances, increased heart rate, anxiety, dependency.

11. **Alcohol** (excessive consumption): Liver damage, addiction, increased risk of certain cancers.

12. **Highly Processed Snacks** (chips, cookies, sugary snacks): Weight gain, dental problems, increased risk of chronic diseases.

Certainly, here are some more foods to be mindful of and their potential harmful effects:

13. **High-Fructose Corn Syrup**: Linked to obesity, insulin resistance, and liver damage.

14. **Artificial Food Coloring and Additives:** May cause hyperactivity in children, allergies, and potential carcinogenic effects.

15. **Fried Foods** (deep-fried in unhealthy oils): Increased risk of heart disease, weight gain, and digestive discomfort.

16. **Highly Processed Vegetable Oils** (soybean oil, corn oil): Imbalance of omega-6 to omega-3 fatty acids, inflammation.

17. **Highly Processed Dairy Products** (sugary yogurts, heavily processed cheeses): Digestive issues, potential for added sugars and unhealthy fats.

18. **Artificial Flavors and Preservatives:**

May contribute to allergic reactions, and some preservatives have been linked to health concerns.

19. **Highly Processed Gluten-Free Foods** (often contain excessive sugar and additives): Lack of nutrients, potential for unbalanced diet.

20. **Highly Processed Vegan Alternatives** (some may be high in additives and preservatives): Nutrient deficiencies, potential for high sodium content.

21. **Excessive Consumption of Red Meat:** Linked to increased risk of heart disease and certain cancers.

22. **Unregulated Herbal Supplements:** Contamination, potential for interactions with medications.

23. **Non-Organic Foods with High Pesticide Residue:** Potential long-term health risks associated with pesticide exposure.

24. **Highly Processed Plant-Based Meat Alternatives:** Some may be high in sodium, additives, and may lack essential nutrients.

25. **Excessive Consumption of High-Mercury Fish** (like shark, swordfish, king mackerel) Mercury toxicity can lead to neurological issues.

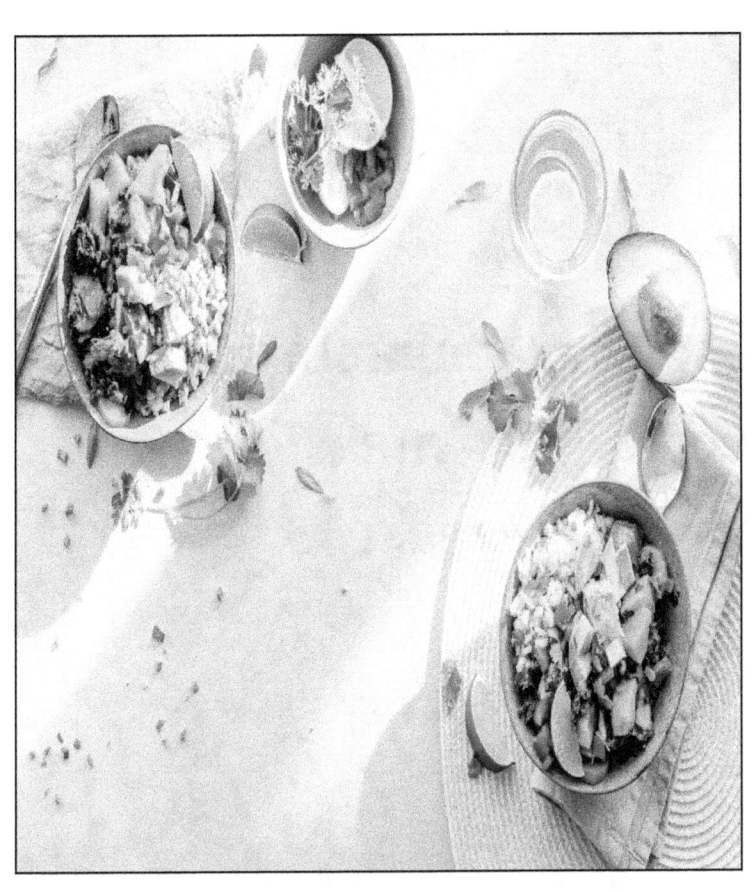

CHAPTER 5:
RECIPES FOR KIDNEY HEALTH

30 KIDNEY-FRIENDLY RECIPES ALONG WITH THEIR PREPARATIONS.

1. GRILLED LEMON HERB SALMON

INGREDIENTS:

- 4 salmon fillets

- 2 tablespoons olive oil

- 1 lemon, sliced

- 2 cloves garlic, minced

- 1 teaspoon dried dill

- Salt and pepper to taste

INSTRUCTIONS:

1. Preheat grill to medium-high heat.

2. In a bowl, combine olive oil, lemon juice, garlic, dill, salt, and pepper.

3. Place salmon fillets on a sheet of foil. Drizzle with the marinade and top with lemon slices.

4. Wrap the foil around the salmon and grill for about 15 minutes, or until cooked through.

2. VEGETABLE STIR-FRY

INGREDIENTS:

- 2 cups mixed vegetables (e.g., bell peppers, broccoli, carrots, snap peas)

- 2 tablespoons low-sodium soy sauce

- 1 tablespoon olive oil

- 2 cloves garlic, minced

- 1 teaspoon ginger, grated

INSTRUCTIONS:

1. Heat olive oil in a large skillet or wok over medium-high heat.

2. Add garlic and ginger, cook for 30 seconds.

3. Add mixed vegetables and stir-fry for about 5 minutes, or until tender-crisp.

4. Stir in soy sauce and cook for an additional 1-2 minutes.

3. QUINOA AND BLACK BEAN SALAD

INGREDIENTS:

- 1 cup quinoa, rinsed

- 2 cups water

- 1 can (15 oz) black beans, drained and rinsed

- 1 cup corn kernels (fresh or frozen)

- 1 red bell pepper, chopped

- 1/4 cup fresh cilantro, chopped

INSTRUCTIONS:

1. In a saucepan, bring water to a boil. Add quinoa, reduce heat, cover, and simmer for 15 minutes. Let cool.

2. In a large bowl, combine quinoa, black beans, corn, bell pepper, and cilantro.

3. Toss with your choice of vinaigrette or lime juice.

4. BAKED CHICKEN WITH SWEET POTATOES

INGREDIENTS:

- 4 boneless, skinless chicken breasts

- 2 medium sweet potatoes, peeled and cubed

- 2 tablespoons olive oil

- 1 teaspoon dried rosemary

- Salt and pepper to taste

INSTRUCTIONS:

1. Preheat oven to 375°F (190°C).

2. Place chicken breasts and sweet potatoes in a baking dish.

3. Drizzle with olive oil, sprinkle with rosemary, salt, and pepper.

4. Bake for about 30-35 minutes, or until chicken is cooked through and sweet potatoes are tender.

5. MUSHROOM AND SPINACH OMELETTE

INGREDIENTS:

- 4 large eggs

- 1/4 cup milk

- 1 cup mushrooms, sliced

- 1 cup fresh spinach leaves

- 1/4 cup shredded low-fat cheese

- Salt and pepper to taste

INSTRUCTIONS:

1. In a bowl, whisk eggs and milk together. Season with salt and pepper.

2. Heat a non-stick skillet over medium heat. Add mushrooms and cook until browned.

3. Add spinach and cook until wilted.

4. Pour egg mixture into the skillet, sprinkle cheese on top, and cook until set.

6. LENTIL AND VEGETABLE SOUP

INGREDIENTS:

-   1 cup green or brown lentils, rinsed

-   6 cups low-sodium vegetable broth

-   2 carrots, chopped

-   2 celery stalks, chopped

-   1 onion, chopped

-   2 cloves garlic, minced

-   1 teaspoon dried thyme

-   Salt and pepper to taste

INSTRUCTIONS:

1. In a large pot, combine lentils, vegetable broth, carrots, celery, onion, garlic, and thyme. Bring to a boil, then reduce heat and simmer for about 30-40 minutes, or until lentils are tender.

2. Season with salt and pepper to taste.

7. TURKEY AND VEGGIE SKEWERS

INGREDIENTS:

- 1 pound turkey breast, cut into cubes

- 1 zucchini, sliced

- 1 red bell pepper, cut into chunks

- 1 red onion, cut into chunks

- 2 tablespoons olive oil

- 1 teaspoon dried oregano

- Salt and pepper to taste

INSTRUCTIONS:

1. Preheat grill to medium-high heat.

2. Thread turkey, zucchini, bell pepper, and onion onto skewers.

3. In a small bowl, combine olive oil, oregano, salt, and pepper. Brush mixture onto skewers.

4. Grill for about 10-15 minutes, or until turkey is cooked through.

8. BROWN RICE AND VEGETABLE STIR-FRY

INGREDIENTS:

- 2 cups cooked brown rice

- 2 cups mixed vegetables (e.g., broccoli, carrots, snow peas)

- 2 tablespoons low-sodium soy sauce

- 1 tablespoon sesame oil

- 2 cloves garlic, minced

- 1 teaspoon ginger, grated

INSTRUCTIONS:

1. In a large skillet or wok, heat sesame oil over medium-high heat.

2. Add garlic and ginger, cook for 30 seconds.

3. Add mixed vegetables and stir-fry for about 5 minutes, or until tender-crisp.

4. Stir in cooked brown rice and soy sauce. Cook for an additional 2-3 minutes.

9. BAKED COD WITH TOMATO AND OLIVE SALSA

INGREDIENTS:

- 4 cod fillets

- 2 tomatoes, diced

- 1/4 cup black olives, sliced

- 1/4 cup fresh basil, chopped

- 2 tablespoons olive oil

- Salt and pepper to taste

INSTRUCTIONS:

1. Preheat oven to 375°F (190°C).

2. Place cod fillets in a baking dish.

3. In a bowl, combine tomatoes, olives, basil, olive oil, salt, and pepper. Spoon mixture over the cod.

4. Bake for about 15-20 minutes, or until fish is cooked through.

10. CHICKPEA AND SPINACH CURRY

INGREDIENTS:

- 2 cans (15 oz) chickpeas, drained and rinsed

- 2 cups fresh spinach leaves

- 1 onion, chopped

- 2 cloves garlic, minced

- 1 can (15 oz) diced tomatoes

- 1 can (15 oz) coconut milk

- 2 tablespoons curry powder

- Salt to taste

INSTRUCTIONS:

1. In a large skillet, sauté onion and garlic until softened.

2. Add chickpeas, diced tomatoes, coconut milk, curry powder, and salt. Simmer for about 15-20 minutes.

3. Stir in spinach and cook until wilted.

11. GRILLED EGGPLANT AND TOMATO STACK

INGREDIENTS:

- 1 large eggplant, sliced

- 2 tomatoes, sliced

- 1/4 cup fresh mozzarella cheese, sliced

- 2 tablespoons olive oil

- 2 tablespoons balsamic vinegar

- Fresh basil leaves for garnish

INSTRUCTIONS:

1. Preheat grill to medium-high heat.

2. Brush eggplant slices with olive oil and grill for about 3-4 minutes per side, or until tender.

3. Assemble stacks by layering eggplant, tomato, and mozzarella. Drizzle with balsamic vinegar and garnish with basil leaves.

12. SPINACH AND FETA STUFFED CHICKEN BREAST

INGREDIENTS:

- 4 boneless, skinless chicken breasts

- 1 cup fresh spinach leaves

- 1/2 cup feta cheese, crumbled

- 2 cloves garlic, minced

- Salt and pepper to taste

INSTRUCTIONS:

1. Preheat oven to 375°F (190°C).

2. Flatten chicken breasts with a meat mallet. Place spinach, feta, and garlic in the center of each breast. Fold and secure with toothpicks.

3. Season with salt and pepper. Place in a baking dish and bake for about 25-30 minutes, or until chicken is cooked through.

13. VEGETABLE AND CHICKPEA CURRY

INGREDIENTS:

- 2 cans (15 oz) chickpeas, drained and rinsed

- 2 cups mixed vegetables (e.g., cauliflower, peas, carrots)

- 1 onion, chopped

- 2 cloves garlic, minced

- 1 can (15 oz) coconut milk

- 2 tablespoons curry powder

- Salt to taste

INSTRUCTIONS:

1. In a large skillet, sauté onion and garlic until softened.

2. Add chickpeas, mixed vegetables, coconut milk, curry powder, and salt. Simmer for about 15-20 minutes.

14. GREEK QUINOA SALAD

INGREDIENTS:

- 1 cup quinoa, rinsed

- 2 cups water

- 1 cucumber, diced

- 1 cup cherry tomatoes, halved

- 1/2 cup feta cheese, crumbled

- 1/4 cup Kalamata olives, sliced

- 2 tablespoons olive oil

- 2 tablespoons lemon juice

- Fresh parsley for garnish

INSTRUCTIONS:

1. In a saucepan, bring water to a boil. Add quinoa, reduce heat, cover, and simmer for 15 minutes. Let cool.

2. In a large bowl, combine quinoa, cucumber, tomatoes, feta, and olives.

3. Drizzle with olive oil and lemon juice. Garnish with fresh parsley.

15. BAKED TURKEY MEATBALLS

INGREDIENTS:

- 1 pound ground turkey

- 1/4 cup breadcrumbs

- 1/4 cup grated Parmesan cheese

- 1/4 cup fresh parsley, chopped

- 1 egg

- 2 cloves garlic, minced

- 1/2 teaspoon dried oregano

- Salt and pepper to taste

INSTRUCTIONS:

1. Preheat oven to 375°F (190°C).

2. In a bowl, combine ground turkey, breadcrumbs, Parmesan cheese, parsley, egg, garlic, oregano, salt, and pepper.

3. Shape mixture into meatballs and place on a baking sheet. Bake for about 20-25 minutes, or until cooked through.

16. BAKED EGGPLANT PARMESAN

INGREDIENTS:

- 1 large eggplant, sliced

- 1 cup whole wheat breadcrumbs

- 1/2 cup grated Parmesan cheese

- 2 cups low-sodium tomato sauce

- 1 cup mozzarella cheese, shredded

- 2 tablespoons olive oil

INSTRUCTIONS:

1. Preheat oven to 375°F (190°C).

2. Dip eggplant slices in egg, then coat with a mixture of breadcrumbs and Parmesan cheese.

3. Place coated eggplant slices on a baking sheet, drizzle with olive oil, and bake for about 20-25 minutes, or until golden brown.

4. Layer eggplant, tomato sauce, and mozzarella cheese in a baking dish. Bake for an additional 15-20 minutes, or until bubbly.

17. SHRIMP AND ASPARAGUS STIR-FRY

INGREDIENTS:

- 1 pound large shrimp, peeled and deveined

- 1 bunch asparagus, trimmed and cut into pieces

- 2 cloves garlic, minced

- 2 tablespoons low-sodium soy sauce

- 1 tablespoon olive oil

INSTRUCTIONS:

1. In a large skillet or wok, heat olive oil over medium-high heat.

2. Add garlic and cook for 30 seconds.

3. Add shrimp and cook for about 2-3 minutes per side, or until pink and cooked through.

4. Add asparagus and soy sauce, stir-fry for an additional 2-3 minutes.

18. MEDITERRANEAN CHICKPEA SALAD

INGREDIENTS:

- 2 cans (15 oz) chickpeas, drained and rinsed

- 1 cucumber, diced

- 1 cup cherry tomatoes, halved

- 1/2 cup feta cheese, crumbled

- 1/4 cup Kalamata olives, sliced

- 2 tablespoons olive oil

- 2 tablespoons lemon juice

- Fresh parsley for garnish

INSTRUCTIONS:

1. In a large bowl, combine chickpeas, cucumber, tomatoes, feta, and olives.

2. Drizzle with olive oil and lemon juice. Toss to combine. Garnish with fresh parsley.

19. LEMON HERB BAKED CHICKEN

INGREDIENTS:

- 4 boneless, skinless chicken breasts

- 2 tablespoons olive oil

- Juice of 2 lemons

- 2 cloves garlic, minced

- 1 teaspoon dried rosemary

- Salt and pepper to taste

INSTRUCTIONS:

1. Preheat oven to 375°F (190°C).

2. In a bowl, combine olive oil, lemon juice, garlic, rosemary, salt, and pepper.

3. Place chicken breasts in a baking dish, pour the marinade over them, and bake for about 25-30 minutes, or until cooked through.

20. VEGETARIAN CHILI

INGREDIENTS:

- 2 cans (15 oz) kidney beans, drained and rinsed

- 1 can (15 oz) black beans, drained and rinsed

- 1 can (15 oz) diced tomatoes

- 1 cup corn kernels (fresh or frozen)

- 1 onion, chopped

- 2 cloves garlic, minced

- 2 tablespoons chili powder

- Salt to taste

INSTRUCTIONS:

1. In a large pot, combine kidney beans, black beans, diced tomatoes, corn, onion, garlic, chili powder, and salt. Simmer for about 20-30 minutes.

CONCLUSION:

A JOURNEY TO VIBRANT RENAL HEALTH

In conclusion, the voyage towards vibrant renal health is a testament to the power of proactive self-care and informed decision-making. Through a balanced diet, regular exercise, and attentive hydration, individuals can fortify their kidneys and pave the way for a flourishing life. Routine check-ups and consultations with healthcare professionals serve as crucial compass points in this journey, ensuring early detection and effective management of any potential issues. Embracing a holistic approach to well-being, encompassing both physical and mental aspects, further solidifies the foundation of robust renal health. Remember, this expedition is not a solitary endeavor; support from loved ones, and the broader medical community, plays an indispensable role. Together, we navigate the currents towards vibrant renal health, unlocking a brighter, more fulfilling future.

As we forge ahead on this path to vibrant renal health, it is essential to acknowledge the significance of perseverance and dedication. Small, consistent steps towards maintaining a kidney-friendly lifestyle can yield monumental results. Each wholesome meal, every mindful sip of water, and every instance of physical activity contributes to the overall well-being of our kidneys.

Furthermore, the importance of awareness cannot be overstated. Understanding the signs and symptoms of renal distress empowers us to take swift action, potentially averting more serious complications. Regular screenings and consultations with healthcare providers remain pivotal in this ongoing journey.

In this pursuit, we also recognize the vital role of research and medical advancements. The relentless dedication of scientists and healthcare professionals in the field of nephrology continually expands our understanding of renal health, leading to innovative treatments and therapies.

Together, as individuals and as a community, we can foster an environment that nurtures and safeguards our kidneys. Let us remain steadfast in our commitment to vibrant renal health, for it is the cornerstone of a flourishing and fulfilling life. With each passing day, we stride closer towards a future where robust kidney function is a shared reality for all.